IRRITABLE BOWEL

SYNDROME TREATMENT

Irritable Bowel Syndrome Treatment

How To Cure Irritable Bowel Syndrome Symptoms

Linda Chung

TABLE OF CONTENT

When You Have IBS

Irritable Bowel Syndrome (IBS) is a serious condition that you must take note of. It is a condition where the bowel isn't functioning as it should. Once diagnosed with these symptoms, the patient would be faced with tremendous pain. If you are yet to be diagnosed by a doctor, you need to head to one immediately.

This book would assist you with understanding what IBS is if you are unable or unwilling to see a doctor. After reading this book, you would be able to decide the effects of IBS on your body and why seeing a doctor can highly increase your chances of curing it, once and for all.

The main problem that many IBS medication is that they aren't safe and have many harsh side effects. Many patients want to know how to safely manage the symptoms of IBS but aren't sure about it. Some others want to live a normal life but find it hard because of the pain associated with these symptoms.

The most difficult part about IBS is that those people who suffer from this condition rarely like to talk about it. It makes sense actually. Who among us like to discuss about our bowels? It's certainly not something you bring up during dinner.

However, you need not worry. There are many great ways that you can use to relieve the pain and uncomfortable feeling caused by IBS. From this book, you would be able to know how to manage your IBS symptoms.

According to a research done, IBS is a condition which affects about fifty percent of those people who visit the gastroenterologist every year. If you feel like you have the symptoms of IBS, do head for someone straight away.

It is highly likely that this condition would create a great amount of pain and discomfort. As such, you need to learn all that you can about your bowels and this illness. That is the main aim of this book. By the end of this book, hopefully you would be able to cure yourself from IBS.

What Is IBS

IBS, or more commonly called as spastic colon to doctors, happens when an individual feels pain in their abdomen. This pain is because of a disorder in the functioning of the bowel and you would also experience changes in your normal bowel habits.

The symptoms of IBS are multiple. When you learn about it, you are better able to understand what is wrong. IBS symptoms may seem like just normal bowel problems, but they are other problems that you need to look out for. Among other symptoms you need to be aware of include having pain in your lower abdomen and stomach bloating.

These symptoms are very important towards deciding if you have IBS or not. Some other common symptoms may also include diarrhea or constipation. For some individuals, it moves from an extreme to another.

However, IBS isn't just limited to such symptoms. You may also have conditions like chronic fatigue syndrome, chronic pelvic pain and stress. There has even been a research which managed to draw a link between having mental conditions and IBS. According to that research, IBS affects both your neurology and psychology.

What Should You Do

Upon realizing that you suffer from IBS, you should find for a relief immediately. The most important thing firstly is to make sure that you have a doctor to diagnose you. Many doctors are able to provide you with the right testing to evaluate your condition.

The doctor would want to track your bowel movements. This would normally be over a certain period and would monitor your other conditions during this period. Among the things that they would look at include:

- Whether or not, you feel relieved from the pain after you have been defecated.

- Is there a change in your stool frequency the moment you feel the pain?
- Is the form or way your stool looks different?

From here, the doctor would decide on the differences and decide whether your condition is normal or not. These conditions are when you have an abnormal condition:

- When you have more than three bowel movements a day or less than thee a week.
- When you have any sign of mucus.
- When you have hard or lumpy stool or a very loose and watery stool.
- When you are straining or an urgent need to go or an inability to finish.

- Feeling of pain in the abdomen or stomach bloating.

Your doctor would most probably do blood work on you as part of the diagnosis process. From there on, he/she would perform a thorough examination on you.

The examination is beneficial in checking out your physical condition. From there, the doctor would be able to rule out other illnesses one by one and come to a conclusion if you are really suffering from IBS.

However, many times, the doctor may not actually find that you have IBS. Several symptoms may indicate that you have some other problems rather than IBS. They include stool, fever, diarrhea or weight loss.

These are all common indications that you face something other than IBS.

Cause Of IBS

There are no conclusive researches for the known cause of IBS yet. Many people who suffer from it have no idea if anyone in their family has it. This could be because it wasn't something that is commonly discussed or that IBS isn't known to be hereditary.

However, you need not worry. The IBS condition is pretty well known that you can find a powerful solution for your pain and discomfort.

Common Treatments Of IBS

There are no hundred percent cures for IBS yet. I doubt there ever be. In most cases, both you and the doctor would need to work on how to handle the symptoms that arise. Without understanding the cause, there is very little that you could do to remove the pain and discomfort.

Another thing you should be aware of is that IBS isn't a condition which progresses over time. You wouldn't suffer more from it than you already have. Besides, it isn't life-threatening unlike other conditions. You shouldn't believe that your pain is fatal and something that you wouldn't be able to cure once and for all.

There are many things that you could do to ensure that your quality of life is maintained. Once you are able to manage those symptoms, you are guaranteed to feel better over the long term.

When it comes to managing IBS, there are many considerations that you need to make. There are certain solutions that you could get from home-remedies, medications and other habits that you can form to stop the pain and subsequent suffering that arises from it.

In many cases, you are able to be relieved just by implementing a single form of treatment. However, many people that suffer from IBS would consider doing more than adding a treatment to their IBS management regimen. You would be able to find multiple benefits from it.

Common Treatments

There are multiple treatments for IBS relief. We would consider the factors in the subsequent chapters. From there, you can slowly adapt it to your lifestyle to provide you with the relief that you need. Among the common reliefs include:

- A Diet Change
- Dealing Better With Stress
- Preventative Measures
- Self-Care Measures
- How To Cope With The Conditions
- Medications
- Herbal Medications
- Complementary Treatments

You should consider each avenue thoroughly if you want to overcome IBS over the long term. Besides, you should also consider the severity of your condition.

If you suffer in a more extreme manner, you would need more help that those suffering from the common IBS. Depending on the severity, you need to ensure that you get the right treatment.

What's Next?

The doctor would diagnose you and decide the severity of your condition. Remember that the severity for IBS is different for everyone. You would need to constantly meet up with your doctor and follow up from his/her diagnosis.

However, you can help the doctor know more about your condition as well. By monitoring your condition levels on your own, you would know better about your condition. The moment you are clear about how severe your condition is, you are better able to use the right tools to cure yourself.

If upon diagnosis, you find that you have mild IBS, you would need to find out what causes it. Work through the stress factors and make the right changes to your diet and common lifestyle habits.

If you suffer from a more moderate condition, you need to make the changes like when you suffer from a mild one with other additional changes. You would need to increase your fiber supplements and possible medications. Be sure to see a doctor to ensure that you take the right kind of medications according to your needs.

If you suffer from a more severe form of IBS, you need to take all the same measures of the mild and severe IBS recommendations, plus also talk to your doctor. Your doctor would prescribe stronger medications.

These stronger medications are important because they are able to control the pain. It is also very helpful to start a journal to note down the pain that you experience on a regular basis. This helps the doctor to understand the pattern of your pain.

What Should You Do?

When sufferers of IBS look for advice about dealing with the problem, I often give the same answer. Make sure that you talk to your family doctor. If your family doctor finds it hard to diagnose your problem, than you should seek a specialist in the field.

Through a series of thorough examination, the doctor would be able to understand better the condition that you face, together with the severity of your symptoms. When this is done, they would be able to give you the right advice that would change your illness over the long term. Most of the time, medications would also be prescribed.

However, it should be noted that seeing a specialist in IBS is the best thing you can do if you are seeking a faster cure. The specialist would guide you by providing you with the proper treatment for your condition.

Nevertheless, you still need to ensure that you are updated about your condition. It is also highly recommended to educate you more about IBS. When you better understand the situation, you would undoubtedly find the relief you desire.

From the next few chapters, you would learn step by step methods towards managing your IBS condition. You would need to consider making the significant difference to the severity of your IBS symptoms, together with the frequency. As you spend your time improving your lifestyle and diet, you would undoubtedly find a relief for your IBS condition.

However, you need to make sure that you see a specialist for the medication chapter. This is because every medication may not suit everyone.

Understanding The Stress Factor

The main thing that many doctors would bring up is stress. Stress is a main factor when it comes to IBS. Stress can damage many aspects of your health, IBS included.

From the beginning, you need to be clear that stress isn't just the main issue. Most of the time, stress is commonly due to multiple factors.

The more stress you put into your body or your psyche, the less healthy you are. Although we aren't too clear about what actually causes IBS, we will need to cure the symptoms that come with it over time. However, stress is normally a main factor.

The Danger Of Stress

All around the world, stress has become a main problem that doctors face. The effect it creates on IBS is also clear.

In an ideal situation, stress is controlled by the body. There is a pain inhabitation system in your bdy which would turn on when it struggles with pain. However, what has been found in patients with IBS is that the hypersensitivity in the body doesn't go away. Your body isn't able to turn on the pain inhabitation system and as such you feel the muscles in your gut hurting.

When you are stressed, you would feel it difficult to relax. When you eat a meal, you would feel that ache in your abdomen that comes with IBS.

Although this would be normal feeling of being full for most people, the people who suffer from IBS would feel the pain. The body isn't able to turn off the pain function. This is different from a common healthy body. As such, you would generally feel more pain.

It May Not Be The Food

The most common misconception is that the pain that you have from IBS comes solely from the food. This isn't very accurate. As a matter of fact, there have even been studies that have been done to confirm this.

Your body experiences a very normal emotional response when you are in the IBS condition. In most people, the emotional reaction isn't something that is just strictly emotional. Your body reacts in multiple ways.

When you feel afraid, nervous or sad, your body reacts physically and emotionally as well. Your heart would start to race, your hands would become sweaty and you would need to use the bathroom constantly.

In most IBS patients, the symptoms would intensify for the stomach pain. We are clear from here that the body reacts to emotional feelings. When you are faced with stressful situations, there would be a prolonged pain in the walls of your stomach. Your gut may be hurt to the point where it would be very difficult for you to move around.

From these, you can be clear that no matter what stress that you place on your body, it can make your symptoms far more painful that the ordinary norm. Your IBS is made more severe from such stresses. Because of this, you need to avoid stressful situations. It would help reduce the number of painful situations.

Of course, it would be highly unlikely that you can avoid all the stress in life. However, you need to remember the impact that stress plays in your IBS condition. It may be very difficult to avoid stressful situations, but you need to learn how to do the things that would make your body cope better with it.

There are two main things that you can do to find relief. From here, you need to take action.

Stress Removal

It is a real challenge for anyone to remove stress from their lives. Without a doubt, everyone would face stressful situations no matter what we try to do to avoid them.

One of the main things to do is to try to relieve you of stress and not to avoid it altogether. When you start relieving yourself of stress, your IBS symptoms would be less likely to pop up.

It is clear that the IBS reaction arises because of the piling of stress. The accumulation of stress over time creates this IBS reaction. To relieve yourself of stress, there are certain measures you can take, among them include:

Avoidance: This remains the best course of action. However, it may not seem very practical at times. If you job is creating a lot of stressful problems for you, consider changing to a different job that you would be able to relax and have more time to unwind. Dealing with bosses and other people can be very difficult and stressful at times.

Meditation: This is perhaps the greatest way for stress relieved. Multiple researches has shown that meditation has the great ability for being able to provide a more relaxed mind. It will provide a better relief from the stressful events that happen in your life. You can even try yoga if you want.

Exercise: Regular exercise has the ability to make you not only healthier, but your body could also relax over time. This is one of the best methods for stress reduction. Try to go for a simple walk every day after dinner. You could even sign up for a membership at the local gym. When you are fit, you are able to perform tasks more efficiently, thus reducing your stress over the long term.

Sleep Well: We often underestimate the power of sleep. Sleep has the amazing ability that helps us recover from our daily activities and recharges us. For good health, good sleep is an absolute must. When you get enough sleep, you would feel rested throughout the day, and you will feel better able to cope with the daily stresses.

Have Fun: Like it or not, difficult situations happen from time to time. This is life. However, you can always look for fun things to do. From watching movies with your friends to going out for drinks with them, this would all help you take the stress away. Everyone need to relax once in a while.

From here, it is clear that stress reduction is a powerful method to avoid IBS. Without a doubt, having the right physical and emotional condition would let your feel better and go through the day dealing with stress better. This in turn, helps you deal with the IBS symptoms better.

Using these methods would help you reduce your stress tremendously. However, there are other ways as well. You would need to find for something that suits you. Changing your environment also helps. Many times, the reason why you are stressed is because you are stucked in a stressful environment. Always remember that stress isn't the only thing you need to consider. We would look into the other chapters in the future chapters.

How Your Diet Affects IBS

Similarly to stress, your diet isn't a main cause of IBS. Many people presume that their condition is caused by eating unhealthy food, but it is certainly not the case for IBS. Although food affects your bowels to a certain extent, it isn't the main cause of your IBS problems.

Food has several problems. Your body would generally react to certain foods more intensely when you have IBS than other people would generally react to. For example, if you suffer from IBS and take some spicy curry, the reaction it causes on your stomach would be different compared to someone who doesn't have IBS.

Additionally, your body would experience an increased level of intestinal muscle reaction when you have IBS. The eating just brings up the symptoms that are already in your bowels. It is not because of the food you take, but your reaction to it.

Food Problems

You can control what you eat. As such, you would be able to control how your body reacts to certain symptoms. Some foods are generally problematic when you have IBS.

This may include alcohol, caffeine or fried foods. Generally most people with IBS would find themselves having a bowel reaction to these foods. Besides, problems can also arise when one person takes too much food.

Some of the IBS sufferers would have diarrhea or cramping in your abdomen because of some sugars that they would find hard to digest. They may include sweeteners in dietetic food, chewing gums and other candies. The general consumption of such sugars would lead to bowel inability to absorb them correctly and lead to diarrhea over the long term.

You would even face certain gas symptoms from time to time. It is commonly brought about by certain food.

Food like beans, legumes, cauliflowers, cabbage and broccoli would generally bring about more intense gas symptoms. When you take such food, it would bring about common IBS symptoms like bloating and increased gas.

As such foods are the reason behind the IBS symptoms; you would need to consider how it would affect you. It is very important that you understand that food affects different people in different ways. Because of this, you would need to discover for yourself as to the reasons for this

Track Your Diet

Perhaps one of the most important things to manage your IBS situation is to keep track of your diet. The goal of this is to ensure that you learn what would worsen your symptoms over the long term. Although you may think you know what you're eating, you wouldn't know how it correlates with your IBS symptoms until you keep track of it.

Ideally speaking, you should track for diet for a minimum of three weeks. This means that you must write down whatever you eat. You would also need to monitor how you feel after taking them. If you feel like you have IBS symptoms, do jot it down. Ensure that the time and date of what you eat as well as the symptoms are properly journal.

Having a tracking chart would help enormously. It would help you track the food that you eat every day and you will know better how you feel after and before every meal. When you do this, you would be clearer as to how certain food bring about different IBS symptoms to you.

Eliminate Certain Food

You tracking chart plays an important role in determining the sort of food which brings problems to your bowel. The moment you find such food, you need to eliminate it completely.

That's the importance in using a chart to track the food you take. You would be better able to decide what affects your bowels and about how to eliminate the right food from your diet. However, many individuals find it hard to cut out certain food from their diets. This is a common problem because they are afraid that they wouldn't be able to enjoy life like they used to have.

Therefore, you could always perform a trial period. Try eliminating those foods that has been known to cause problems to you and see if you are able to cure your IBS symptoms over the long term. If you still can't, then perhaps taking that food doesn't matter in the first place.

When you eliminate food from your diet, may cause additional problems as well. When individuals remove too many foods, they are unable to have the sufficient nutrient in their lifestyle. This poses another additional health concern. Certain individuals would then suffer from illnesses such as anemia or nutrient deficiency.

Like it or not, you shouldn't remove entire foot groups. If any diets ask you to do so, avoid them at all costs. There are many diets that ask you to remove all fats or carbohydrates. This is just unhealthy regardless of the short term affects you may get from it. If you use these tracking charts to your benefits, you should only use it with the help of your doctor and their guidance

However, if upon discussion with your doctor, he/she believes that there are certain food which affects you to a certain condition, you would need to perform certain tests. Tests like allergy tests, lactose breathing testing and upper intestinal endoscope are all helpful in determining the condition that you are in.

In certain conditions, your body would have a common intolerance which would make you feel the symptoms of IBS more heavily. Testing would be able to help the doctor determine if you really have them. There are also certain illness that come together with IBS. Among them include:

- **Food Allergy**. This is a response from your immune system to those foods that you are eating.

- **Lactose Intolerance** - A condition that your body isn't able to digest milk.

- **GERD**. Stands for Gastro Esophageal Reflux Disease, a chronic reflux of gases into esophagus.

- **Eosinophili Gastroenteritis**. A rare condition where there is a reaction to food where white blood cells enter the GI tract which causs illness.

Through thorough testing, your doctor would determine if you have these conditions. They would worsen the symptoms that you face with the IBS symptoms.

Be Careful About How Much You Eat

It is also important to keep track about how much you have eaten. As much as the type of food you consume would affect your body, you also need to be clear that the amount of food you eat would also heavily affect your body. Take time to read diet books to learn the right portion that you should take.

When a person has IBS, they shouldn't be consuming too much food in a single sitting. Many Americans aren't aware that they simply eat too much. This doesn't only make them overweight, but creates digestion problems. When you overeat, there is a tendency for your body to be reactive due to IBS.

To ensure that you eat the right amount of food, make sure that you read the packaging label first. This is a way to consider how much food to be taken in a single sitting. With food labels, you are better able to divide the serving size.

These are among the portions that you should be taking when you are monitoring your IBS situation. It is a great estimate to start with.

- Fruit - A cup of fruit should be enough.
- A slice of bread.
- Pasta or Rice. One half cup is a serving.

- Salad - A cup of salad is enough.
- Meats like fish, poultry, beef and pork - three ounces is enough for one serving
- Ice Cream - Half a cup

These are all rough estimates that you could use. As you can see, many of the servings are smaller than how much people eat. That is because most people eat way too much in the first place. Habits are hard to change. But if you change for the better, I'm sure you would be able to get a grip of your IBS condition.

Most people would look at the portion control with anxiety. How could they feed themselves? It seems like the food is way too little for them to be full. It is fully understandable that some people need to eat more.

For example, men need to eat more than women due to their size. Meanwhile, those who exercise more definitely need to eat more. Children and teenagers need to consume more as they are growing.

It is understandable that the portion control may not be practical for some people. Therefore, you may adjust the portions as you deem fit. This all depends on individual. Talk to your family doctor about it.

How To Eat Less?

Many people struggle to eat less because of their bad habits. These are among the best tips that I know that would help you eat less.

- **Eat Slower.** When you eat slower, your body is able to get full faster. Many people eat too fast and fail to realize that they are already full.
- **Pay Attention.** Start to pay attention how much food they are eating. Don't put too much food in your plate in the first place.
- **Use Smaller Plates.** Smaller plates give you the illusion that you eat more already. If you use a larger plate,

there is a tendency to think that you haven't eat enough.

- **Pay Attention To How Much You Eat.** Keep a track record to determine if you are overeating throughout the day.

These tips may seem simple, but they go a long way in changing your health and improving your lifestyle. As you pay more attention to this, you would be able to reduce the amount you eat and the IBS symptoms that come with it.

How Much To Limit Yourself?

Limiting yourself is very difficult to gauge. If you limit yourself too much, it would invariably damage your health over the long term.

However, there is absolutely no need to go on an absolutely strict diet. When you limit yourself strictly, you would eventually fail to follow through on your diet. Diets which are too strict are much harder to follow over the long term.

Besides, it isn't a good idea to completely neglect a good group. Every food has its pros and cons. Therefore, you would need to find out which food brings out the IBS symptoms in you. From there, start to control and limit the intake of food.

You need to realize that a well-balanced diet is very important if you are to live a healthy lifestyle.

You need to learn that there are many strict diets and you don't have to follow it strictly. Unless your doctor says that you have to be strict on it, make it as flexible and fun as you can.

IBS Diet Tips

Understanding what food is right to eat is your responsibility if you want to be cured of IBS symptoms. You need to understand what the best food for you is. Remember that every person experience food differently. Therefore, you need to experiment if these tips are useful for you.

Among the useful tips for IBS patients include:

- Drink Enough Water. Eight cups isn't enough. Go for ten.
- Don't Forget To Eat Fiber.
- Reduce Fatty And Fried Food Consumption.

- Food With Fructose and Sorbitol Should Be Completely Removed From Your Diet.
- Reduce Alcohol And Caffeine Intake.
- Take Six Small Meals A Day, instead of three meals a day.

As you do these entire things, you would be able to improve your diet and your overall health. When you reduce the IBS symptoms, you would definitely feel better. Speaking with your doctor is helpful as he may give you more specific directions.

Importance Of Fiber

Fiber is known to be something good to consume. However those who suffer from IBS need to carefully manage their fiber intake. If you take too much fiber, it would lead to diarrhea. If you take too little, you end up being constipated.

To know the right amount to take, you need to experiment. You would need to first decide by taking a variety of different fibers. Consume fiber from fruits, whole grains and vegetables. These are all natural fiber and are great for your IBS condition.

The body needs fiber to stimulate the colon muscles and soften your stool. The gas produced by fiber helps it to do so.

However, those who suffer from IBS would suffer from several things. When you add too much fiber, there would more discomfort. Because of this, you should deeply monitor the amount of fiber you take each day. The best method to get fiber for those with IBS is to get it from food that has citrus or take legumes.

Food Is Important

You need to be clear that the food you take doesn't cause your IBS problems. They are just the stimulus for how badly your IBS situation has become. As you find out which food causes you to suffer and slowly limit or remove them, you would see a healthier you.

When you eat a more balanced diet and restrict certain foods that aren't helpful to you, you would see those improvements quickly.

IBS Medications

When diagnosed with Irritable Bowel Syndrome, there are many medicinal choices. Those medications aren't normally given to everyone who suffers from IBS but mainly those who suffer from an extreme level of IBS.

This means that for most conditions of IBS, medications may not even be necessary. Those medications come in several forms and you may have heard plenty about them. To choose the right medication for you, you would need to be thorough with your doctor. Your doctor would be able to determine the right medication for you.

If you find a certain medication but your doctor has yet to tell you about it yet, don't take it until you get the advice from your doctor. Always be sure about such things. Because every single situation is different, certain medications may not suit you at all.

Without a doubt, the highest benefit comes not from the medications but from your changes in your lifestyle. You also need to better manage your stress level. The doctor would always prescribe those changes before anything else.

Only after those have failed that you look to use medication. There are several options of medication that you should look for. They would be explained thoroughly in this chapter.

First Line Of Medication

Over-the-counter medications are the first line of medication. In most cases, IBS symptoms are not severe and there would be no need at all for prescription treatment. However, doctors would recommend certain basic medications to protect your body from getting weaker.

One main medication would be anti-diarrhea medication. This medication helps control diarrhea. One most common type is called as loperamide. The brand name is called as Imodium.

The other form of medication that your doctor would prescribe to you would be fiber supplements. Fiber is an important nutrient that helps you maintain your health. When diagnosed with IBS, having the appropriate amount of fiber helps provide relieve in constipation. You can get fiber from supplements pills. Look for Psyllium, under the brand name of Metamucil and methylcellulose, under the brand name of Citrucel.

Prescription Medications

It is clear that there are few options when you want relief for your IBS symptoms. In terms of prescription medications, there are few that are being used which are the same like the first line of medication.

The two main ones are anticholinergic medications and antidepressants.

Anticholinergic medications assist you with the problem with your nervous systems. Some people with IBs would require such medication so that they are able to regulate their nervous system activities. They provide relief from certain spasms pain that arise from your bowel.

Certain people would need antidepressants because of their depression and the pain associated with it. If this is the case, the doctor may assist you with antidepressants or serotonin reuptake inhibitor. These medications help with common depression symptoms, as well as help control the intenstines throughout the neurons in your brain.

You could also work with a counselor or psychiatrist if you feel bouts of depression. It is a very common situation to be depressed. They would be able to give you advice about your mental issues.

Medication Specifically For IBS

Throughout the years of research, there has been many IBS medication which are being produced as well. Those medications may or may not suit you, but it is important that you have a certain idea about what it is.

You need to discuss with your doctor about it to determine if they are the right ones for you to help you relieve your IBS symptoms.

The two main medications being used to treat IBS currently are Alosetron (Lotronex) and Tegaserod (Zelnom).

Alosetron, or under the brand name Lotronex, is something of a controversy. This is because the FDA (Food and Drug

Administration) removed it from the market a few years back. At least two hundred individuals had severe side effects due to this drug and research attributed it to this drug.

However, the FDA decided to allow it into the market again in 2002, bar some restrictions. This medication is used to relax the colon and slow the movement of waste through the lower bowel. It will therefore help relieve the symptoms of IBS.

In today medical condition, this medication is only prescribing to women patients. Besides, only doctors who are specifically trained are allowed to prescribe them. If you doctor prescribe this drug to you, make sure you talk to him clearly about the potential side effects that you could suffer from.

Tegaserod, or under the brand name of Zelnom, is another very common medication. It has been shown to be incredibly effective in managing IBS symptoms.

This drug imitates the action of the neurotransmitter serotonin and helps to get the nerves and muscles in the intestines in the right track and relieves constipation over the long term.

However, it has to be clear that studies have shown that this drug create severe side effects in certain individuals. If you doctor really prescribes this medication, make sure that you monitor for any side effects that you experience. Should anything feel severe, talk to your doctor and stop medication immediately.

Like said before, any form of medication would only be taken after you have made lifestyle changes. This includes changes in your eating habits as well as managing stress in a better way.

Additionally, seeing a specialist helps tremendously if you condition feels like it's getting worst. Please be clear that medication may not be for you. You have other treatments that are freely available for you. This is further discussed in future chapters.

Alternative Treatments

In the past few chapters, we have talked a lot about using medications and making changes to your lifestyle in order to deal with IBS. It is perhaps the most challenging condition to deal with because of the concerns about the various effects of the medications.

However, you need not worry. There are also alternative treatments and herbal remedies that you can try to ensure that you are able to control your IBS symptoms.

Like many alternative treatments, there isn't any guarantee that they would work for you. Certain treatments help some people while it wouldn't help other people.

However, if a certain treatment could help you, there is no harm in trying it. That's a benefit about using alternative treatments, the effects are minimal but the potential long term benefits are huge.

From this chapter, we would share certain alternative treatments that you could try. In many cases you are able to use them with other treatments for extra IBS benefit.

As with many other conditions out there, there are many alternative treatments for IBS too.

From healing a cold to fighting cancer, IBS can be treated with the right alternative treatment too. Alternative treatments are great because of the minimal side effects that you would experience.

Complementary Therapy

When looking for IBS medications, you may want to consider complementary therapy. Complementary treatments refer to medications that could be taken with other medication or lifestyle changes. When in complement, you would have greater chances of improving your IBS symptoms. Among the complementary therapy to consider when fighting IBS include:

- Using Herbal And Dietary Products
- Somatic Therapies
- Breathing And Movement Therapy
- Mind-Body Therapy

These therapies, when used properly, can be extremely beneficial to the patient over the long term. In most cases, there aren't any adverse side effects. The extreme benefit of complementary treatment is that you are able to treat a person in a holistic manner rather than only treating the symptoms that you experience.

In terms of Western medication, there are many people who don't agree with the doctors are the approach given. Therefore, with the use of complimentary treatments allow you the control you need.

In the next few pages, we would understand better the complimentary therapies that you could consider for IBS treatment. Try any of these methods because the side effect is minimal.

Herbal Therapy

This is a form of therapy that is normally found from plants. Plants products help make someone feel better. In most cases, ancient Chinese civilizations are the ones that have influenced the herbal remedies that has spanned over thousands of years. Some therapy works while some don't.

For herbal therapies that deal with IBS, there are normally more than a single set of herbal ingredients or therapy. This is because of the general norm of ancient medication.

Traditional medication doesn't just look at the disease but your health on a whole. Traditional medication is known to be more holistic when dealing with the symptoms.

However, most herbal treatments have been modified because some of those ingredients aren't readily available. To cure IBS, the most common herbs include barley, tangerine peel, rhubarb, cardamom and licorice.

As you purchase the herbs, it is most likely that the herbal product would contain multiple herbs in a single form. Therefore, when you are purchasing those herbs, you need to pay attention to whom you are purchasing them from and product quality. If you don't go for the best quality or the purest form, you would struggle to benefit from the herbs.

Even if you don't really believe in herbal treatments, you have nothing to lose if you try. In fact, research has proved that herbal products are highly effective to curing a person's IBS symptoms. They come back with improved symptoms.

These are among the additional supplements that you could take to provide improvements. These are all herbs based.

- **Ginger** - A common food in IBS symptoms relief. You can use ginger in many ways. You could use ginger extract if you have IBS. Just consuming a few drops daily would go a long way to providing anti-inflammatory condition and improving the quality of your gastric system lining. It would also assist your intestines do a better job.

- **Artichoke Leaf Extract** - This is very common herb that is used in Europe. This would improve in the bile secretion of the sufferer. However, not many studies have been done for this treatment yet.

- **Peppermint Oil** - This is especially great for gastrointestinal conditions. However, you should be aware of the amount of it you take because it may cause you to suffer from heartburns. If consumed moderately, it would be extremely beneficial. It helps decreases the muscle spasm that your GI tract would have to experience. It would also relieve bloating and pain in your abdomen. To take peppermint oil, simply drop a few of it into your drink.

- **Others Herbal Products** - There are many other herbal products to help you. Rhubarb root is especially helpful for constipation. Consuming just a small of such products through supplement pills would greatly assist your constipation relief.

Movement Therapy

Another great IBS therapy is movement therapy. After using this therapy, the individual would be able to use their energy for relaxation and better in dealing with IBS symptoms. Among the best treatments to consider include tai chi and yoga. These therapies would benefit you one way or another. When you start doing it, you would be able to benefit from them over time.

However, such therapy doesn't only help you with your IBS problems. Over the long run such exercises would also help improve your physical and psychological health.

From the previous chapters, I have made it clear that stress reduction is something that you must seriously take into consideration. When you start using these movement therapies, you would be able to change your lifestyle for the better.

You could easily start yoga or tai chi by visiting a local gym. Start up with a beginner's course as this allows you to learn the true form of such exercises. It is also highly recommended that you do it on a consistent basis.

Mind Body Therapy

Without a doubt, there is a big connection between the emotional states that you are in and IBS. When you use mind-body therapy you would slowly improve your overall well-being and reduce the impact of the IBS symptoms. The main therapy is meditation. We have discussed this in the chapters before, but we will go into slightly deeper detail from here.

Meditation is an incredible method to relax your body and let your mind be at ease. When it comes to fighting IBS, meditation is a very important thing if you want to cure it long term. Besides, meditation also allows stress reduction which helps in the IBS symptoms reduction.

If you feel that meditation isn't for you, you could try hypnotherapy. It has been proven to be an excellent tool to reduce IBS symptoms.

Visit a hypnotic professional to ensure that you get the right treatment. To ensure the benefits, hypnosis session should be around once a week. You need to do this over a period of a few months in order to get the best results. In hypnosis, the patient would need to perform progressive relaxation.

When you use hypnosis effectively, you can see several benefits. They may include reductions in abdominal pains, reduce constipation and general improvement in your quality of life.

You need to find a really qualified therapist in order to ensure proper treatment. This is perhaps the most important thing. Another note to consider is that it is perhaps a very expensive method to treat IBS. However, if money isn't really an issue for you, do try it.

Acupuncture

For a few thousand years, acupuncture has been proven to be effective in healing many medical conditions. Regardless of whether you believe it or not, acupuncture works. If something has been alive for so many years, you can be sure that it is effective. Now, it is used around the world and growing more popular by the day.

For those who aren't aware of what acupuncture is, it is based on the channels of energy. These energy channels are called Qi. These energy channel travels through the entire body.

In these energy channels, there are three hundred and sixty different acupuncture points. While you are healthy, the energy in your body flows easily. However, if you aren't healthy, the energy flow would be disrupted. This is a possible reason why you have IBS.

As such, this is the power of acupuncture. It is used at certain locations around your body to release energy and bring back the energy flow in your body.

Acupuncture helps IBS as it would relieve the pain in the abdomen. Through the right channeling of energy, you would be able to relieve nausea and stomach bloating also.

If you would like to try out acupuncture, the most important thing is to find for a very skilled and experienced acupuncturist.

The acupuncturist should have an excellent track record.

Talk to him about your condition and see if he is able to help. Talk to him specifically about your IBS. He may even be able to prescribe herbal remedies.

Using Probiotics

Probiotics work as they alter your intestinal flora and are incredibly helpful in treating IBS. Probiotics are generally organisms that would help regulate bacteria that are in your intestines. When you balance those bacteria, you would be able to benefit from these symptoms for relief.

Intestinal floras are good bacteria that are in your intestines. Its purpose is to ensure that the GI tract works correctly. They are organisms that are throughout your intestines and help make sure that you have a healthy immune system and provide the secretion of fluid.

The logic is such: The natural bacterial benefits could be able to treat IBS as well. Because of this, probiotics is used to simulate the intestinal flora. According to research, it is also extremely beneficial in helping to reduce the amount of pain that someone experiences in the abdomen. This reduction of gas is evident when you use probiotics while for many people, their bowels also tend to function better over time when they use probiotics.

Probiotics can be easily purchases from health food stores. Although there are still studies that are ongoing about the benefits for IBS symptoms control, it is definitely something proven, according to my experience.

Complimentary Therapies For You?

These options depend on the individual suffering from IBS. For many people, they prefer to stick with just traditional medications. For certain other people, the greatest benefit of complimentary therapy is that they would avoid the harmful side effects from the use of medications. This is a decision that you must make.

You need to remember that there are people who use complimentary therapies use it together with both medications and making lifestyle changes as well. However, you must always talk to your doctor about it. You need to find the entire possible cure for your IBS symptoms. This therapy may be just the proper choice, if you give it a try.

IBS Prevention

When it comes to the best IBS medication, the most important thing you could do is prevention. This is perhaps the most important thing. You don't have to think too much about IBS and learn as much as you can. You need to plan before the symptoms come in. As we aren't sure about what causes IBS, you would need to find out first.

To make sure that IBS doesn't happen again, prevention is something that you should definitely always keep in mind. It is generally up to you and what you do when your symptoms arises. As we can't completely cure IBS yet, there are many things to prevent the symptoms from arising. Among the best tools to prevent IBS include:

- **Diet**: You diet is perhaps the most important part. Like I have said in the previous chapters, your diet doesn't cause IBS, but it could trigger it. Improving your diet is perhaps the most important part in IBS prevention. To do this, you have plenty of opportunities to do so. Use the eating journal to decide what you should or shouldn't eat. When you start to know your body better, you can control your diet better. Decide for yourself if you need a more balanced diet or to eliminate more things from your life. Make sure that you also consume the proper amount of fiber. If you are constipated, fiber is incredibly important. You may even need supplements.

- **Exercise**: Your body needs to be physically active and you need to have your exercise daily. This may include brisk-walking to other physical activity. When you are physically active, your body is better equipped to deal with the daily stresses of life. Even the easiest walk in the park can go a long way towards improving your lifestyle. When you start with this habit, you would eventually get used to it.

- **Mind Therapy**: Meditation and counseling are the main things you can do for mind therapy. You can do a lot on your own to reduce and prevent the IBS symptoms that are evident. You wouldn't be able to see the benefits of these therapies immediately, but give it time, and you will be able to see the benefits of it. These mays to relieve stress and relax are incredible. Find time before and after work to relax for a few minutes a day.

- **Counseling**: You need to work with your doctor to plan the right treatment. You should also consider counseling and when it comes to IBS, you need to remember that you are dealing with more than a physical issue. You are also dealing with a psychological and emotional issue. Because of this, you need to consider a psychologist or psychiatrist. As you invest sessions with a psychologist, you would be better equipped to deal with the huge levels of stress that would trigger IBS symptoms. Your counselor could go a long way towards helping your stressful situations.

- **Biofeedback**: Is an excellent technique that you could learn to reduce the amount of stress that you are under. From here, you would learn to accomplish it with a machine. It would help reduce the muscle tension that you feel and slows down your heart rate. Talk to your doctor about it. In many cases, this could be done in your medical center and you would be able to find out more through your local hospital.

- **Hypnosis**: Plays a role in lowering the amount of pain that you feel. When you have a skill hypnotist, you are able to feel more relaxed after hypnosis. From here, you are better able to deal with the symptoms that you face due to IBS. From my experience, there are patients who are able to reduce their pain that comes from their abdomen cramps and stomach bloating. Besides, having a skilled hypnotist would help prevent the onset of symptoms. They would teach you how to deal with them when they come.

- **Deeper Breathing Techniques**: It is without a doubt that your breathing would affect the quality of your life. This is also true for those looking to manage their IBS symptoms. Breathing well (deeper) would be extremely helpful if you face IBS. Most people breathe from their chest. However, you would be better able to relax if you start to learn how to breathe from your diaphragm instead. This quickens your IBS relief as this form of breathing allows you to relax your abdominal muscles, which reduces the strain and pain caused by IBS.

In dealing with IBS, the main goal is to prevent it. If you can't manage to get all the various techniques to help you in your bid to manage the symptoms, look for other methods. I believe that those stress relief methods would definitely do you a lot of good. Make sure that you are constantly relaxed. This will help you feel better and reduce the IBS symptoms.

These changes may feel small, but it can make a lot of difference in your life.

The IBS Checklist

If you have Irritable Bowel Syndrome, you can expect to face it for a few years. As IBS cannot be completely cured, you must expect to deal with it effectively. There are many things you could do to ensure your IBS becomes more manageable.

- **Change Your Diet**. Do according to the recommendations from the beginning of the chapters. Find out the food that worsen your symptoms and remove them.

- **Talk To Your Doctor**. Check if you need medication. You would need more clarification with regards to this because some medication creates side-effects.

- **Consider Alternative Treatment**. Try a few of them and see which one suits you best.

- **Stress Relief**. The best way to relieve stress is prevention. Use the methods prescribed in this book.

- **Keep Educated**. Know about the latest studies and treatment methods of IBS. Look to read more about it. You can even join forums to discuss your problems.

IBS prevention is the key thing to ensure your health is taken care off. Start from the beginning and work your way through them. Change is difficult.

Start your way with a few changes first. From there, you would be better able to improve your lifestyle and the symptoms.

I wish you all the best in your treatment of IBS. With the right mindset, I'm sure you would be able to cope with it easily.

Resource 1 - Natural IBS Cure

Want a natural cure for IBS?

The best cure for IBS is by using natural cures. Natural cures are safe and highly effective... Discover them here...

http://ibsnatural.wellbeingvalley.com/

Resource 2 - IBS Secret Systems

From this guide, you would discover

- **5 Different Tests You Can Perform On Yourself**
- When And How To Use Probiotics
- **Why Vitamins And Minerals Are An Intgral Part of IBS Treatment**
- How To Deal With The 8 IBS Causes
- **11 treatments and self-help For IBS Cure**
- How your immune system could be attacking some of the things you eat.
- **An entire elimination diet with a step-by-step 42 day guide to help you identify if you have any intolerance to certain foods or food groups.**
- How Lectins could be causing havoc on your body – and which foods they're found in.

http://ibssecrets.wellbeingvalley.com/

www.ingramcontent.com/pod-product-compliance
Lightning Source LLC
Chambersburg PA
CBHW070538290526
45790CB00002B/556